SAY NO TO DEATH

100 TIPS TO AVOID EARLY DEATH

INTRODUCTION

Death is indeed inevitable,but guess what,you can live life to it's fullest,if you just follow thses few tips.

Included below are also tips to prevent and treat Suicidal thoughts..

Chapter 1

Housekeeping Clues

1. Try not to remove remains from the chimney or wood oven among Christmas and New Year's Day.

2. Never put a brush on a bed.

3. Close umbrellas prior to bringing them into a house.

4. Try not to clear after twilight.

5. You mustn't wash garments on New Year Day.

6. Try not to shake out a decorative spread into the evening.

7. Never wash a banner.

8. Try not to turn a seat on one leg.

9. Keep felines off piano keys.

10. Try not to drape a dishcloth on a door handle.

11. Clearing under a wiped out individual's bed will kill that person.

12. Never, at any point rock a void recliner.

Remodel and Designing

13. Never add-on to the rear of your home.

14. You mustn't cut another window in an old house; the best way to keep away from deadly outcomes is to throw your cover through the new window, and afterward go through it yourself.

15. Never drive a nail after nightfall.

16. Try not to move into an incomplete house.

17. Try not to convey tomahawks, scoops, and other sharp-edged instruments through a house; in the event that you should accept one inside, consistently take it out by a similar entryway.

18. On the off chance that you move out of a house, don't move once more into it for a year.

19. Try not to hang your darling's image topsy turvy.

20. On the off chance that an image tumbles from the wall, don't get it.

21. Never convey a peacock's plume into a house.

22. Keep cut blossoms out of rooms for the time being.

23. Never convey a bunch of wildflowers inside before May 1.

Sewing and Design

24. In the event that you cut out another dress on Friday, you should complete it that very day.

25. Try not to make new garments among Christmas and New Year's Day.

26. Never hold a stick in your mouth while sewing.

27. Continuously sew cross-sewing on your clothing.

28. Try not to stroll around in one shoe.

29. On the off chance that you see a will-o'- wisp while out strolling around evening time, turn your jacket back to front.

30. Never wear one more's new garments before they have worn them.

31. A lady who makes her own wedding dress won't live to wear it.

Cooking and Social graces

32. Never set three lights on a table simultaneously.

33. Try not to set the table in reverse.

34. Never serve 13 at a table.

35. Try not to drink espresso at 5 o'clock.

36. You mustn't compose on the rear of a dish.

37. Never return acquired salt.

38. Never cross blades while preparing the table.

39. Be certain that another person prepares your birthday supper.

40. Try not to put two forks at one spot setting.

41. Never, never flip around a portion of bread.

Resting

42. Laying down with your head at the foot of the bed is certainly deadly.

43. Try not to sing in bed.

44. On the off chance that you hear a canine yell around evening time, arrive at under the bed and turn over a shoe.

45. Try not to count stars.

46. A man ought to never dream of an exposed lady; a lady ought to never dream of a bare man. (You know what your identity is...)

Individual Cleanliness

47. Never rub cleanser on your skin on a Friday.

48. Try not to investigate a mirror behind another.

49. Try not to brush your hair into the evening.

50. Positively no hair styles in Spring.

51. Let a child's hair and fingernails develop until their first birthday celebration.

52. Try not to allow two individuals to brush your hair immediately.

53. Never shave around evening time.

54. Never under any circumstance share a razor utilized by a dead man.

Burial service Decorum

55. Never hold a burial service on a Friday.

56. At the point when an individual passes on in a house, you should promptly cover all mirrors and shut down all clocks.

57. Youngsters shouldn't profess to have burial services.

58. Never take a stab at a grieving cloak.

59. Continuously eliminate a dead body from a house feet first.

60. Never ride in a funeral car, except if you are the driver.

61. Try not to include the vehicles in a burial service motorcade.

62. Try not to wear new garments to a burial service, particularly new shoes.

63. Pull the shades in a room where a burial service is occurring; in the event that the sun hits a griever's face, he is the close to pass on.

64. While strolling in a memorial service parade, don't look in reverse.

65. Never point at a grave.

66. Do whatever it takes not to step across a grave.

67. Never leave a grave open for the time being.

68. Never be quick to leave the cemetery after a burial service. (Also, trust that not every other person observes this guideline, as well...)

69. On the off chance that a carcass lies unburied on Sunday, one more around will clearly kick the bucket soon.

70. Stand by a year prior to setting up a gravestone for a relative; in the event that you don't, another relative will go before the year has finished.

General and Different

71. Drink May water.

72. At the point when debilitated, don't search in mirrors.

73. Try not to give an individual a peony.

74. Never measure your own level.

75. Do whatever it takes not to envision it's Saturday when it's not.

76. Try not to count vehicles on a traveler train.

77. Never whistle in a coal mineshaft.

78. Abstain from estimating an individual who is resting.

79. Try not to walk in reverse.

80. You mustn't permit a flame to wear itself out.

81. Never sell a canine.

82. Do whatever it takes not to kill a crow; but rather in the event that you do, make certain to cover it while sporting dark.

83. On the off chance that you relocate a cedar tree, you will bite the dust when concealing a grave is sufficiently large.

84. The equivalent is valid for a willow tree (as in 83)

85. Never balance your digger on a tree limb.

86. Try not to skirt a line while establishing corn or beans.

87. In the event that you watch an individual carefullyconcealed, you'll at no point ever see them in the future.

88. Abstain from venturing over an individual who is resting.

89. At the point when your name is called, don't answer the initial occasion when it very well might be Satan calling you.

90. Never shake hands through a window or over a wall.

91. Do whatever it takes not to sit with your back to the fire.

92. Try not to consume sassafras wood.

93. Assuming you stroll with your hands locked behind your head, it will kill your mom.

94. Don't Consider taunting an owl. (Who?)

95. Try not to store your shoes over your head.

96. Never kill a beetle.

97. Never kill a reptile.

98. On the off chance that you hear a hen crow, you should kill the hen.

99. On the off chance that you are on a train when a lady sheets, wearing dark, get off.

100. Anything you do, don't allow a reptile to count your teeth. (Truly, simply DON'T.)

Chapter 2

Risk factors for early passings for our ages.

It found that the most widely recognized risk factors for sickness and early demise are like those until the end of the Australian populace, which include:

Tobacco smoking

Hypertension

High blood cholesterol

Weight

Unreasonable liquor utilization

Actual latency.

Tobacco smoking

Tobacco smoking is a critical gamble factor for different malignant growths (like cellular breakdown in the lungs), persistent obstructive pneumonic sickness and cardiovascular illness. Research recommends that smoking was answerable for around 10% of all cardiovascular passings all through the world in 2000.

In the event that you smoke, stop in a hurry.

Look for proficient guidance assuming you find it hard to stop. Meanwhile, attempt to scale back. Research recommends that the gamble of malignant growth, coronary illness and respiratory sickness is portion related, and that implies the gamble expands the more cigarettes you smoke. Nonetheless, that doesn't mean there is a protected degree of smoking.

Hypertension

Hypertension (hypertension) can cause ischaemic coronary illness (impeded courses in the heart), stroke, hypertensive coronary illness, fringe vascular sickness and renal (kidney) disappointment.

Lose overabundance weight.

Do more actual work - in a perfect world, something like 30 minutes consistently.

Eat all the more new leafy foods.

Diminish or take out dietary salt - lessening your salt admission by 3g each day brings down pulse, however the impact is multiplied with a 6g each day decrease and significantly increased with a 9g each day decrease. A low-salt eating regimen likewise diminishes your gamble of cardiovascular sickness.

Barbara J Smith

High blood cholesterol

Cholesterol is a fat-like substance tracked down in the circulation system. Factors, for example, heredity, an eating routine high in soaked fat and different circumstances, for example, type 2 diabetes impact an individual's cholesterol level. High blood cholesterol might demolish atherosclerosis (restricting of the veins) and impact the improvement of coronary illness and stroke.

Diminish how much immersed fat (the fat from creature items) in your eating routine.

Increment utilization of new organic product, vegetables and wholegrain cereals.

Consume one to two serves of fish each week, especially sleek fish. Concentrates on show that around 100g each seven day stretch of sleek fish - like salmon - lessens the gamble of death from coronary illness by 34% and is defensive against coronary illness and stroke.

Heftiness

In 2009, close to half of grown-up Victorians were classified as overweight or large. Inordinate muscle to fat ratio conveys a higher gamble of chronic sickness including coronary illness, stroke, type 2 diabetes, colon malignant growth, nerve bladder infection and osteoporosis. Being overweight is additionally connected to hypertension and high blood cholesterol.

Shed pounds with quality food decisions and customary activity.

Plan to shed pounds steadily, as crash consumes less calories don't work and may try and make you put on more weight over the long haul.

Look for proficient guidance from your primary care physician or dietitian on the off chance that horrible weight demonstrates troublesome.

Unreasonable liquor utilization

Unreasonable long haul drinking builds the gamble of malignant growths of the mouth, pharynx, throat and liver. Smoking and unreasonable liquor exacerbates things. Tobacco smoking intensifies the disease causing impacts of liquor on the upper intestinal system and respiratory plot. Liquor is likewise connected to viciousness and an expanded gamble of unplanned injury.

Stay away from hitting the bottle hard - that is, drinking a lot of liquor in a solitary meeting.

Put forth a cognizant attempt to diminish your drinking - for instance, before you go to a café supper, settle on a set number of beverages (like two) and stick to it.

Diminish your admittance to liquor - for instance, don't store mass sums at home.

Trade between cocktails and non-cocktails - water is great - when you are drinking.

Change to drinks with a diminished liquor content in the event that you would be able - for instance, drink light lager rather than original capacity brew.

Drink wine rather than spirits like bourbon - spirits are refined instead of matured and have a lot higher liquor content.

Go for the gold two liquor free days consistently.

Actual idleness

On the off chance that you are not dynamic, your gamble of cardiovascular illness is expanded, particularly coronary illness. Overweight and stout individuals are likewise prone to be inactive.

Do a sensible measure of activity no less than multiple times every week ('sensible' signifies sufficiently to make you puff and sweat).

Pick a game or movement you appreciate, on the grounds that the 'fun component' emphatically expands your inspiration to work out.

Get going gradually in the event that you are not used to ordinary activity - increment the recurrence and force as your wellness moves along.

Make a point to check with your PCP before you start any new activity program - individual factors, for example, your age or a prior ailment could make a few types of activity improper or even unsafe.

Where to find support

Your primary care physician

Your neighborhood local area wellbeing focus

Things to recall

You can decisively lessen your gamble of early demise by simplifying a couple of way of life changes.

The most widely recognized reasons for sickness and sudden passing in our age incorporate tobacco smoking, hypertension, high blood cholesterol, weight, over the top liquor utilization and actual idleness.

Being a non-smoker, eating a sound eating routine, practicing consistently and restricting liquor utilization can decrease your gamble of numerous possibly deadly illnesses like coronary illness, stroke and malignant growth

Conclusion

Your PCP might do an actual test, tests and top to bottom addressing about your psychological and actual wellbeing to assist with figuring out the thing might be causing your self-destructive reasoning and to decide the best treatment.

Appraisals might include:

Psychological well-being conditions. Much of the time, self-destructive considerations are connected to a basic emotional wellness issue that can be dealt with. If so, you might have to see a specialist who works in diagnosing and treating psychological sickness (therapist) or other emotional wellness supplier.

Actual medical issue. Now and again, self-destructive reasoning might be connected to a hidden actual medical issue. You might require blood tests and different tests to decide if this is the situation.

Liquor and medication abuse. For some individuals, liquor or medications assume a part in self-destructive reasoning and finished self destruction. Your PCP will want to find out whether you generally dislike liquor or medication use —, for example, gorging or being not able to scale back or stopped utilizing liquor or medications all alone. Many individuals who feel self-destructive need treatment to assist them with halting utilizing liquor or medications, to diminish their self-destructive sentiments.

Drugs. In certain individuals, certain remedy or non-prescription medications can cause self-destructive sentiments. Inform your primary care physician regarding any prescriptions you take to see whether they could be connected to your self-destructive reasoning.

Kids and youngsters

Kids who are feeling self-destructive typically need to see a therapist or clinician experienced in diagnosing and treating youngsters with emotional wellness issues. Notwithstanding persistent conversation, the specialist will need to get a precise image of what's rolling on from various sources, for example, the guardians or gatekeepers, others near the kid or adolescent, school reports, and past clinical or mental assessments.

Treatment

Treatment of self-destructive considerations and conduct relies upon your particular circumstance, including your degree of self destruction chance and what fundamental issues might be causing your self-destructive contemplations or conduct.

Chapter 3

Suicide and Suicidal Treatment

Nonemergency circumstances

On the off chance that you have self-destructive considerations, yet aren't in an emergency circumstance, you might require short term treatment. This treatment might include:

Psychotherapy. In psychotherapy, additionally called mental advising or talk treatment, you investigate the issues that cause you to feel self-destructive and master abilities to assist with dealing with feelings all the more really. You and your specialist can cooperate to foster a treatment plan and objectives.

Prescriptions. Antidepressants, antipsychotic prescriptions, against uneasiness meds and different meds for psychological sickness can assist with diminishing side effects, which can assist you with feeling less self-destructive.

Fixation treatment. Treatment for medication or liquor fixation can incorporate detoxification, enslavement treatment projects and self improvement gathering gatherings.

Family backing and instruction. Your friends and family can be both a wellspring of help and struggle. Including them in treatment can assist them with understanding what you're going through, give them better adapting abilities, and further develop family correspondence and connections.

Helping a friend or family member

In the event that you have a friend or family member who has endeavored self destruction, or on the other hand in the event that you figure your cherished one might be at risk for doing as such, get crisis help. Try not to let the individual be.

On the off chance that you have a friend or family member you think might be thinking about self destruction, have a transparent conversation about your interests. You will most likely be unable to compel somebody to look for proficient consideration, yet you can offer consolation and backing. You can likewise help your cherished one track down a certified specialist or psychological well-being supplier and make an arrangement. You might actually propose to come.

Supporting a friend or family member who is persistently self-destructive can upsetting and exhaust. You might be apprehensive and feel remorseful and powerless. Exploit assets about self destruction and self destruction avoidance with the goal that you have data and devices to make a move when required. Additionally, deal with yourself by getting support from family, companions, associations and experts.

Way of life and home cures

There's not a viable replacement for proficient assistance with regards to treating self-destructive reasoning and forestalling self destruction. Notwithstanding, there are a couple of things that might lessen self destruction risk:

Stay away from medications and liquor. Liquor and sporting medications can deteriorate self-destructive contemplations. They can likewise cause you to feel less restrained, and that implies you're bound to follow up on your viewpoints.

Structure areas of strength for an organization. That might incorporate family, companions or individuals from your congregation, temple or other spot of love. Strict practice has been displayed to assist with decreasing the gamble of self destruction.

Get dynamic. Actual work and exercise have been displayed to decrease sadness side effects. Consider strolling, running, swimming, cultivating or taking up one more type of actual work that you appreciate.

Adapting and support

Try not to attempt to oversee self-destructive contemplations or conduct all alone. You really want proficient assistance and support to beat the issues connected to self-destructive reasoning. Furthermore:

Go to your arrangements. Try not to skip treatment meetings or regular checkups, regardless of whether you need to go or don't feel like you want to.

Accept prescriptions as coordinated. Regardless of whether you're feeling great, don't skirt your drugs. In the event that you stop, your self-destructive sentiments might return. You could likewise encounter withdrawal-like side effects from unexpectedly halting an upper or other drug.

Find out about your condition. Finding out about your condition can enable and inspire you to adhere to your treatment plan. Assuming you have despondency, for example, find out about its causes and medicines.

Focus on cautioning signs. Work with your primary care physician or specialist to realize what could set off your self-destructive sentiments. Figure out how to detect the peril signs early, and conclude what moves toward take somewhat early. Contact your primary care physician or specialist assuming that you notice any progressions by they way you feel. Consider including relatives or companions in looking for advance notice signs.

Make an arrangement so you understand what to do on the off chance that self-destructive considerations return. You might need to settle on a composed concurrence with a psychological well-being supplier or a friend or family member to assist you with expecting the right moves toward take when you don't have the best judgment. Obviously expressing your self-destructive expectation with your specialist makes it conceivable to expect it and address it.

Take out possible method for committing suicide. In the event that you figure you could follow up on self-destructive contemplations, quickly dispose of any possible method for committing suicide, like guns, blades or perilous drugs. On the off chance that you take prescriptions that have a potential for glut, have a relative or companion give you your drugs as endorsed.

Look for help from a care group. Various associations are accessible to assist you with adapting to self-destructive reasoning and perceive that there are numerous choices in your day to day existence other than self destruction.

Planning for your arrangement

At the point when you call your essential consideration specialist to set up an arrangement, you might be alluded quickly to a specialist. In the event that you're at risk for committing suicide, your primary care physician might have you get crisis help at the medical clinic.

What you can do

Make these strides before your arrangement:

Make a rundown of key individual data, including any significant burdens or late life altering events.

Make a rundown of all prescriptions, nutrients and different enhancements that you're taking, and the dosages. Be straightforward with your primary care physician about your liquor and medication use.

Inquire as to whether conceivable — somebody who goes with you might recall something that you missed or neglected.

Make a rundown of inquiries to pose to your primary care physician.

A few essential inquiries to pose to your primary care physician include:

Might my self-destructive considerations at some point be connected to a hidden mental or actual medical issue?

Will I really want any tests for conceivable basic circumstances?

Do I want quick treatment or the like? What will that include?

What are the options in contrast to the methodology that you're proposing?

I have these other mental or actual medical conditions. How might I best oversee them together?

Is there anything I can do to remain safe and feel much improved?

Would it be a good idea for me to see a specialist?

Is there a nonexclusive option in contrast to the medication you're endorsing me?

Are there any pamphlets or other literature that I can have? What sites do you suggest?

Make sure to extra inquiries.

What's in store from your primary care physician

Your primary care physician is probably going to pose you various inquiries, for example,

When did you initially start having self-destructive considerations?

Have your self-destructive considerations been ceaseless or incidental?

Have you at any point attempted to end your own life?

Do you have an arrangement to commit suicide?

In the event that you have an arrangement, does it include a particular strategy, spot or time?

Have you made any arrangements, for example, gathering pills or composing self destruction notes?

Do you feel like you have some control over your motivations when you want to kill or harming yourself?

Do you have companions or relatives you can converse with or go to for help?

Do you drink liquor, and assuming this is the case, how much and how frequently?

What meds do you take?

Do you utilize sporting medications?

What, regardless, assists you with managing your self-destructive contemplations?

What, regardless, seems to demolish your self-destructive contemplations?

What are your sentiments about what's in store? Do you have any expectation that things will get to the next level?

Getting ready and expecting questions will assist you with taking full advantage of your experience with the specialist.

What you can do meanwhile

In the event that you've planned an arrangement and can't see your PCP right away, ensure you stay safe. Contact relatives, companions or others you trust to help you. In the event that you feel you're at risk for harming yourself or endeavoring self destruction, call 911 or get crisis help right away.

www.ingramcontent.com/pod-product-compliance
Lightning Source LLC
LaVergne TN
LVHW020544160826
845677LV00015B/4185

* 9 7 9 8 3 5 1 9 9 7 2 6 1 *